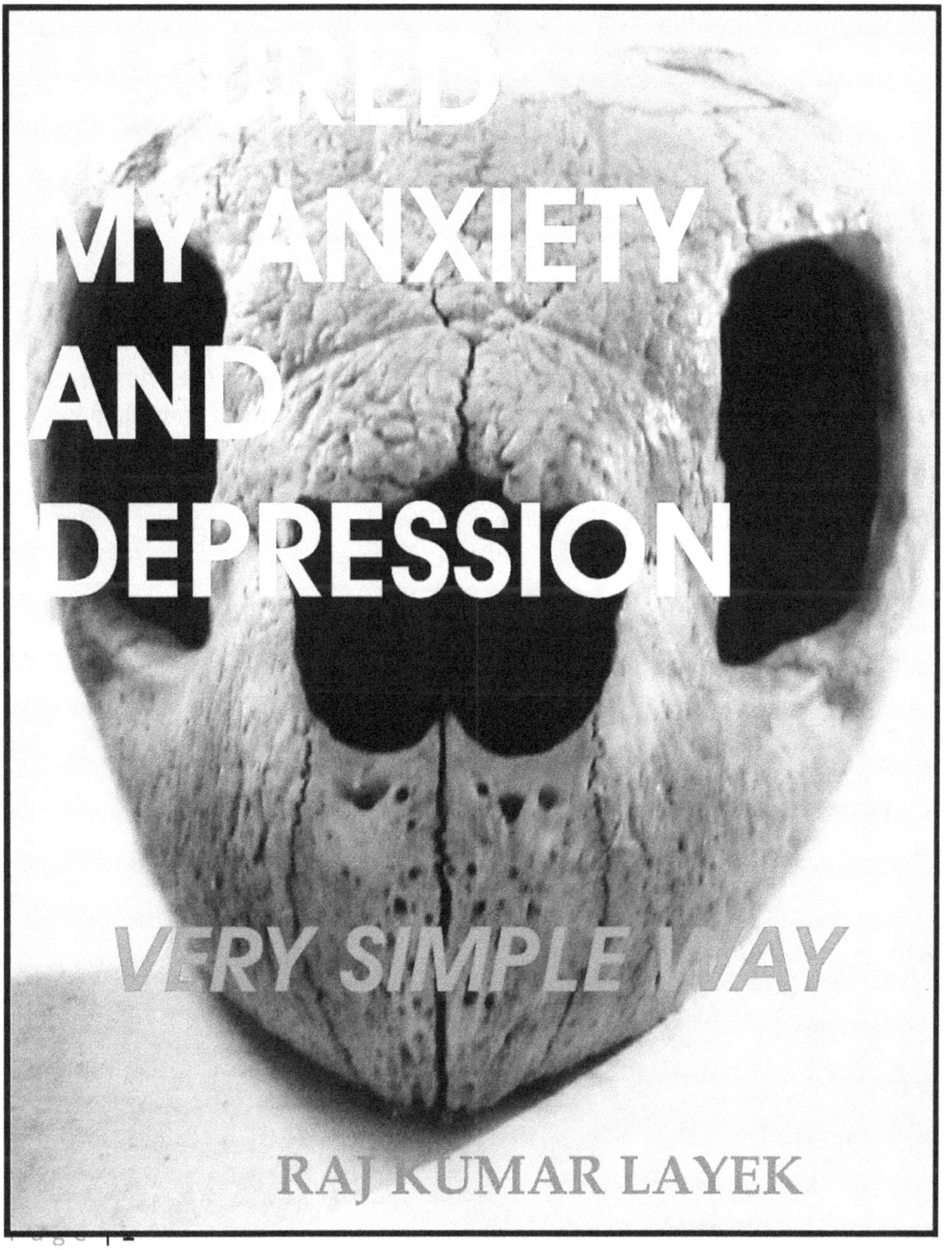

CURED

MY ANXIETY
AND
DEPRESSION

VERY SIMPLE WAY

RAJ KUMAR LAYEK

I CURED MY ANXIETY AND DEPRESSION

RAJ KUMAR LAYEK

Copyright © 2017 RAJ KUMAR LAYEK

Front cover image by Auther.

Book design by Auther.

DEDICATION

This book is dedicated to all fighters who fight against the anxiety and

depression.

TABLE OF CONTENTS

Author's Note

This book is a product of my personal journey. Within its pages, I share the methods and techniques that I personally employed to overcome anxiety and depression. Every method and approach I discuss has been something I've tried and found effective in my own quest for healing. Rather than creating an extensive and lengthy book filled with unnecessary details, I've chosen to distill the essential information. I understand that those dealing with anxiety and depression may not have the patience to sift through a long book, searching for key insights.

This book is designed for efficiency. You can read through it in just 30 to 40 minutes without losing your focus or patience. The goal is to help you find the important information you need without getting lost in unnecessary details. By following the crucial instructions provided within, you can complete the book quickly and then embark on the journey to improve your condition. If you diligently apply the recommended techniques, you might even notice positive results or changes within just a week. My intention is that this book fulfills its purpose of offering practical guidance to those seeking relief from anxiety and depression.

ACKNOWLEDGMENTS

I gratefully acknowledge and express deep appreciation to my family members, my elder sister, sister and brother.

CHAPTER ONE 1:

WHAT IS IT?

"The more you try to impress, the more you become depressed, and the more they get tired of your coercion. It doesn't make them love you, instead, they'll see you as a little child, trying to draw a senseless picture on a piece of paper, begging people to look at it and admire it by force. You can persuade someone to look at your face, but you can't persuade them to see the beauty therein."................. – Michael Bassey Johnson

WHAT IS IT?

Anxiety and Depression:

Anxiety and depression can be likened to the experience of "living in a hell." It's a state where you're aware of what you should be doing, the rules you should be following, and your own shortcomings, yet an overpowering force within you prevents you from engaging in positive actions. You feel weak, timid, and helpless, observing your own challenging circumstances. There's a part of you that yearns to break free, but you often find yourself retreating to a comfort zone that isn't truly comfortable, yet feels familiar. This creates a sense of hopelessness that permeates your being.

Personally, I struggled with anxiety, agoraphobia, depression, the fear of falling ill suddenly while traveling, vertigo, and gradually developed hypochondria. These challenges stole five precious years of my life (though they also imparted valuable life lessons). My journey led me to visit numerous doctors, counselors, and try various medications they prescribed, but the tormenting feelings kept returning with even greater strength. Despite facing these adversities, I managed to excel in the first three semesters of my M.Sc. program. However, the final semester proved to be more difficult, causing a decline in my performance. This led to a loss of my university's gold medal, which I had previously been on track to receive. Fortunately, my brother was in the same department and his companionship helped me complete my M.Sc.

Subsequently, I found myself in a condition unfit for pursuing a Ph.D. I became confined to my home, predominantly to my bed, spending my days watching television. With each passing day, my situation deteriorated further.

If you're reading this book, you're likely familiar with the intricate details of these struggles. The most challenging aspect is that you're unable to articulate these feelings to your family, friends, children, spouse, or even medical professionals.

One day, I came across an advertisement for the State Forest Service Exam, sparking a desire within me to join the service. This ignited a sense of frustration towards my own condition. I made a commitment to transform myself and started contemplating potential solutions. It became evident that the erroneous signals and information I was receiving were stemming from my brain, leading to a deficiency in essential chemicals like dopamine. This realization prompted me to provide my mind and brain with the necessary nutrients and habits to facilitate healing. Through consistent efforts, I managed to alleviate nearly 90% of my condition within a year and a half.

While it might appear that this period is an extended duration for overcoming such challenges, I discovered that rushing the process often results in setbacks. The timeline is dependent on the severity of the issue and the determination to heal.

CHAPTER TWO 2:

HOW IT DEVELOPED?

"What lies behind us, and what lies before us, are tiny matters compared to what lies within us."—Ralph Waldo Emerson

HOW IT DEVELOPED?

The emergence of my anxiety and depression wasn't sudden; it gradually developed over time due to various factors. There was a starting point to this journey. During my years in college from 2003 to 2006, I didn't experience any significant fear, anxiety, or depression while traveling alone. However, this changed after witnessing a series of terrifying accidents on the National Highway during trips from my hometown to the capital city. I was a frequent traveler, often visiting various places, particularly my ancestral village.

After completing my graduation, I began preparing for competitive services, particularly the banking sector. This phase led me to confine myself to a room for study and practice. Over time, I realized that I started avoiding going outside. Initially, I considered this mentality helpful for my studies, but it was a mistake.

My initial mistake was reducing interaction with friends and avoiding social gatherings. This withdrawal was detrimental to both my mental health and physical well-being.

The second mistake was isolating myself from friends. It's important to have supportive friends who reduce stress and negativity.

Neglecting proper nutritious food was another mistake I made.

Recognizing the importance of sunlight for mood improvement came later. I had developed a habit of studying late at night and sleeping during the day, which deprived me of necessary sunlight exposure.

I realized that LED lights, especially before sleep, were disruptive to proper sleep. I also had the habit of browsing the internet at night, which affected the quality of my sleep.

Engaging with social media before sleep had an adverse impact, inducing feelings of emptiness and unhappiness, especially while battling anxiety and depression.

In search of solutions for my general health issues, I developed the habit of self-diagnosing through internet research. However, this tendency created unnecessary worry, as I constantly felt unwell and convinced myself I had various ailments.

The entire experience can be summarized using the words of the renowned writer Jerome K. Jerome from "Three Men in a Boat (To Say Nothing of the Dog)":

"I remember going to the British Museum one day to read up the treatment for some slight ailment of which I had a touch—hay fever, I fancy it was. I got down the book and read all I came to read; and then, in an unthinking moment, I idly turned the leaves, and began to indolently study diseases, generally. I forget which was the first distemper I plunged into—some fearful, devastating scourge, I know—and, before I had glanced half down the list of 'premonitory symptoms,' it was borne in upon me that I had fairly got it. I sat for a while, frozen with horror; and then, in the listlessness of despair, I again turned over the pages. I came to typhoid fever—read the symptoms—discovered that I had typhoid fever, must have had it for months without knowing it—wondered what else I had got; turned up St. Vitus's Dance—found, as I expected, that I had that too, began to get interested in my case, and determined to sift it to the bottom, and so started alphabetically—read up ague, and learnt that I was sickening for it, and that the acute stage would commence in about another fortnight. Bright's disease, I was relieved to find, I had only in a modified form, and, so far as that was concerned, I might live for years. Cholera I had, with severe complications; and diphtheria I seemed to have been born with. I plodded conscientiously through the twenty-six letters, and the only malady I could conclude I had not got was housemaid's knee. I felt rather hurt about this at first; it seemed somehow to be a sort of slight. Why hadn't I got housemaid's knee? Why this invidious reservation? After a while, however, less grasping feelings prevailed. I reflected that I had every other known malady in the pharmacology, and I grew less selfish, and determined to do without housemaid's knee. Gout, in its most malignant stage, it would appear, had seized me without my being aware of it; and zymosis I had evidently been suffering with from boyhood. There were no more diseases after zymosis, so I concluded there was nothing else the matter with me."

Today, searching the internet for potential illnesses is easy, with millions of pages on symptoms available. This habit can be detrimental to a healthy mind, resembling slow poison. Gradually, I began to believe I had various ailments, eventually developing hypochondria.

Therefore, I strongly advise the following:

Refrain from filling your mind with unfamiliar information.
Avoid searching for symptoms of potential diseases.
Avoid sleeping with the TV on, especially tuned to negative news channels.
Our subconscious mind absorbs surrounding influences during sleep, affecting our mental state.

One day, the intensity of my condition grew stronger than I could have imagined.

CHAPTER THREE 3:

UNDERSTANDING THE PROBLEMS

"Understanding is the first step to acceptance, and only with acceptance can there be recovery."
— J.K. Rowling, Harry Potter and the Goblet of Fire

UNDERSTANDING THE PROBLEMS:

Initially, I assumed that my struggles were temporary and would naturally fade over time. However, my persistence in maintaining detrimental habits related to my anxiety and depression prevented any spontaneous improvements. My comfort zone became a prison, eliminating any hope for automatic progress.

Although my siblings frequently advised me to take deliberate steps towards healing and growth, I resisted leaving my comfort zone. Despite lacking the mental strength for a complete transformation, I was aware that changing my thinking patterns and lifestyle held the key to improvement—just as you might recognize too.

One day, an advertisement for a forest ranger officer job caught my attention. This government job posed a significant challenge, with a stringent selection process that included a physically demanding walking test of 25 km in 4 hours. Despite the obstacles, I was determined to succeed in this role. To begin, I meticulously assessed my problems.

I recognized, through modern medical science, that I had no underlying health issues. My hypochondria led me to undergo numerous tests, all of which yielded results that a healthy person would receive. This realization led me to adopt the mantra: "Why Worry?"

A substantial phobia of traveling alone posed a major barrier to success.

A prolonged lack of preparation for the job instilled a fear of losing out on the opportunity, but I began adopting a positive perspective, reminding myself that I had ample time for proper preparation.

A lack of self-confidence also hindered my progress.

By jotting down these issues, I gained clarity. What initially appeared to be an insurmountable challenge was narrowed down to three core problems, with the second issue being particularly significant.

Intrigued by my own circumstances, I delved into understanding the root of my phobia for traveling alone. Many people encountered similar experiences while traveling daily or frequently. Yet, they didn't succumb to fear. Numerous individuals drove cars, trucks, and buses regularly, witnessing similar incidents, but they didn't develop a phobia like I did.

A sudden realization struck me: it was my brain that had been sending me erroneous signals about the outside world, activating panic responses unnecessarily. My brain's neurons weren't functioning like those of others. Moreover, my brain wasn't producing adequate amounts of dopamine, a chemical responsible for feelings of happiness.

This prompted another question: why was this happening? I concluded that my brain's neurons lacked essential nutrients required for optimal performance.

My search led me to explore books and resources detailing methods for improvement. I sought to determine which foods, habits, and exercises were beneficial for brain health and neuron function. I worked diligently to cultivate a positive outlook on life.

During this exploration, I came across the concept of neuroplasticity. A book on the subject enlightened me about the existence of a neural loop in the brain. This loop triggered anxiety by perceiving potential threats and unnecessarily preparing the body for emergencies, even in the absence of actual danger. This loop had been formed by my thoughts about the road accident during travel.

To break this anxiety loop, I realized I needed a robust mindset, a positive attitude, refusal to entertain negative thoughts about travel, and positive self-suggestions. This approach yielded remarkable results, emphasizing the powerful interplay between the mind and the brain.

Book: The power of neuroplasticity by Shad halsteller.

CHAPTER FOUR 4:

JOURNEY TO CHANGE

"The beautiful journey of today can only begin when we learn to let go of yesterday." — Steve Maraboli, Unapologetically You: Reflections on Life and the Human Experience

JOURNEY TO CHANGE:

The path to transformation was far from easy, yet my determination to change remained unyielding. It's a well-known truth that change and improvement often come hand-in-hand with discomfort. While recognizing that our present circumstances might be more agonizing than the potential for progress, we still cling to our comfort zones, allowing space for fear and anxiety to fester.

My self-created comfort zone exhibited several traits:

I began to settle for compromises.
I became enslaved by my own mind.
Above all, I succumbed to the allure of constant sleep. Initially, this tactic provided some relief, but over time, my sleep patterns deteriorated until I found myself in a state of perpetual wakefulness—days and nights blurred into a disorienting haze akin to a person bitten by a snake who then gets hit by a car on the way to the hospital.
However, I was resolute in my quest to transform myself. Amid the endless cycle of thought and the struggle to initiate change, a beacon appeared in the form of the book "POWER OF NOW." This serendipitous encounter marked the moment when I ceased incessant contemplation.

Actions commenced:

Recognizing the detrimental impact of TV, I discontinued its consumption.

Morning routines embraced yoga, and within days, positive results surfaced.

Initial improvements yielded a measure of confidence.

Incorporating a daily regimen of seeds and herbs became a norm:

Ocimum sanctum: daily
Bacopa monnieri: daily
Centella asiatica: after a few days, eventually daily
(Caution: These herbs are potent. While you can consume one leaf daily on an empty stomach, be prepared for potential initial reactions.)
Acquiring a manual treadmill proved to be transformative. Though I initially lacked the power and patience for an extended walk, I gradually built up from 5 to 10, 20, and then 30 minutes. This exercise not only instilled newfound confidence but also alleviated anxiety. Furthermore, it catalyzed an improvement in appetite, digestion, and overall bodily strength. Enhanced digestion maximized nutrient absorption, which positively impacted my well-being. This newfound vitality emboldened me to venture outside.

The boundaries of my comfort zone began to expand. Short trips to the local grocery and sweet shops became part of my routine. Walking with my brother around our neighborhood in a 1- to 2-kilometer loop bolstered my confidence. During these walks, I discovered the transformative power of music to elevate my mood, enhancing my overall experience.

I embarked on a journey of solitude by sitting alone for gradually increasing durations in the mornings. This practice fostered confidence through measured exposure to the outside world.

Another effective technique materialized: before sleep, I'd recline on my bed, deliberately relaxing each body part, clearing my mind of distractions, and embracing concrete suggestions for improvement.

Mornings emerged as a period of rapid development for enhancing my condition. I adhered to certain principles:

I shunned negative self-suggestions.

I learned the value of patience, allowing my mind to clear.

Mindfulness of breath allowed my mind to tranquillize.

Nighttime meditation encouraged self-suggestion.

To curb racing thoughts, I tuned into songs in languages I didn't understand, such as Russian and Telugu. This technique redirected my brain's attention, minimizing the emergence of anxiety-inducing thoughts.

Language learning unexpectedly proved valuable. At a time when I had halted job preparation, I turned to Sudoku puzzles and a Japanese-learning app. My commitment to Sudoku fueled patience, perhaps spurred by a sibling rivalry. This experience illuminated the efficacy of mild competition in motivating tasks. Learning a new language, as per a newspaper article, promised to enhance brain power. Embracing this advice, I began using Duolingo to learn Japanese.

CHAPTER FIVE 5:

IDENTIFYING FAULTS AND IMPLEMENTING CORRECTIONS

"A man must be big enough to admit his mistakes, smart enough to profit from them, and strong enough to correct them"………John C. Maxwell

IDENTIFYING FAULTS AND IMPLEMENTING CORRECTIONS:

Realizing that mere reading and noting down remedies wouldn't be enough, I understood that practical implementation of suitable methods for physical and psychological improvement was essential. This realization marked my initial fault. To rectify this, I embarked on various methods that could enhance my physical strength, mental well-being, and overall confidence.

My second fault was failing to sustain consistency. Within a week, my motivation dwindled, causing me to abandon strenuous activities like exercise, walking, and yoga. However, I persisted with methods related to dietary habits and herbal remedies due to the firm guidance of my elder sister, who closely supervised this aspect.

Addressing this fault, I eventually managed to adhere to a regular exercise and yoga routine. Overcoming inconsistency is challenging, and if you also struggle with it, remember that it's common for those dealing with depression and anxiety. The key is never to give up entirely. Restart promptly, whether there's a gap or your mind insists you're faltering.

My third fault emerged from comparing myself with others. Witnessing their engagement in work, play, and travel, I felt inadequate and burdened by immense tension. I eventually stopped such comparisons, realizing that challenges are nature's way of guiding us toward better paths or aligning us with our life goals.

Fourthly, as I began recovering from my challenges, I became a zealous advocate of positive thinking and other strategies. However, I soon learned that advising others while still struggling was counterproductive.

It negatively impacted my belief system, especially when pessimistic individuals disregarded my advice and contributed doubt.

UNDERSTANDING THE WORKINGS OF MY MIND

My mind played intriguing games with me, often sabotaging my efforts. It fed me excuses, such as believing that merely possessing knowledge of an effective method equated to implementing it. It tempted me to delay actions, promising I could start tomorrow, and as a result, I never initiated anything.

This deceptive mental dance continued until I recognized its pattern. My inner self intervened, reminding me that the path of improvement required consistent effort, not mere intention. I used the analogy of smoking and cancer to emphasize that good habits, unlike addictions, don't provide immediate gratification. Despite knowing this truth, I struggled to follow it.

My inner voice grew assertive, asserting that I was the master of my mind, not the other way around. This declaration led to a nightly ritual of planning the next day's activities. This agreement between my conscious self and my wandering mind facilitated adherence to routines.

Upon joining a strict service environment, I adhered to routines imposed by external authority. I recognized that even if my mind resisted, I could rely on discipline to carry me through. The transformation demanded persistence, commitment, and an understanding of my mind's tricks.

CHAPTER SIX 6:

GRATITUDE

"Always have an attitude of gratitude."......... Sterling K. Brown

GRATITUDE :

Amidst my struggles, I often found myself waiting, hoping for someone to acknowledge my efforts with gratitude. However, I came to understand that proactively expressing gratitude yields far more satisfaction than waiting for it from others. This expression doesn't always involve monetary assistance; it could be in the form of kind words, empathy, or small sacrifices that make a notable impact.

The Benefits of Demonstrating Gratitude to Others

Enhanced Confidence: Engaging in acts of gratitude boosts your self-assurance. It empowers you to move beyond self-pity and showcases your quality of character.

Karmic Reciprocity: Displaying gratitude may eventually yield direct or indirect rewards, but it's essential not to expect anything in return from those you've helped. Expectations can turn genuine gratitude into a transactional barter system.

Divine Endowment: Gratitude illustrates that you possess a positive trait bestowed by a higher power, suggesting you are capable of enriching the lives of those around you.

Nurturing Relationships: Expressing gratitude cultivates a circle of good friends and well-wishers who might offer valuable advice and caution against unwise decisions in various aspects of life.

Divine Alignment: Those who consistently express gratitude often experience a sense of divine alignment in their lives. This alignment could manifest in various forms of positivity.

Enhanced Well-being: The act of gratitude contributes to overall well-being, particularly on the psychological front, by fostering a positive mindset and emotional equilibrium.

Incorporating gratitude into your life offers a myriad of advantages beyond receiving acknowledgment from others. It empowers you, nurtures connections, and positively impacts your overall health and outlook.

CHAPTER SEVEN 7:

SUCCESS CANNOT BE DUPLICATED, BUT IT CAN BE ATTAINED.

"However difficult life may seem, there is always something you can do and succeed at." – Stephen Hawking

SUCCESS CANNOT BE DUPLICATED, BUT IT CAN BE ATTAINED.

In a historical academy dedicated to ranger training, our additional director imparted a thought-provoking lesson: "Success cannot be replicated but can be achieved." At first glance, this statement may seem contradictory, particularly in the context of his lecture on global forest protection and conservation efforts. However, he illuminated the idea by emphasizing that success stories cannot be blindly transplanted from one setting to another due to the intricate interplay of social structures, environmental conditions, and cultural beliefs that differ across regions.

Reflecting on my own journey, I recognize that attempting to directly emulate various success stories led to challenges. While these stories certainly provided valuable lessons, I lacked the realization that "THE SUCCESS CANNOT REPLICATE BUT CAN BE ACHIEVED."

Upon closer examination, I've discerned some critical points:

Diverse Social Structures: The structure of society varies greatly across different regions. For instance, in many Western countries, individuals typically live independently from their families after reaching adulthood. Contrastingly, in India, it is customary for families to remain closely interconnected and provide mutual support. This distinction profoundly influences how success is pursued and understood.

Cultural Beliefs: Personal beliefs and cultural norms shape perspectives on success. As an Indian following Hindu beliefs, I find solace in the notion of rebirth and the eternal nature of the soul. This belief system bolsters my resilience, but it also carries the potential risk of fostering complacency, as some may become overly reliant on the prospect of a better life in a future incarnation.

Environmental Impact: The environment profoundly affects physical and mental well-being. The pace of recovery for someone dwelling by a serene forest differs significantly from that of an individual living in a bustling, polluted city.

Nutritional Choices: The role of diet in health is widely acknowledged. It is crucial to identify and eliminate foods that undermine well-being and instead embrace those that promote vitality.

In essence, while learning from the experiences of others is invaluable, it is essential to adapt these lessons to one's unique circumstances. The path to success is multifaceted, woven with the threads of individuality, culture, environment, and personal beliefs. Rather than seeking a direct replica of another's triumph, we must weave our tapestry of achievement, harmonizing these elements into a vibrant mosaic that reflects our own journey and aspirations.

CHAPTER EIGHT 8:

WHAT HAD I LEARNED DURING MY TRAINING?

"Tell me and I forget, teach me and I may remember, involve me and I learn."……… Benjamin Franklin, Founding Father of the United States

WHAT HAD I LEARNED DURING MY TRAINING?

During my range officer training, I came to realize the ease of adhering to routine under authority. The experience of strict discipline at the Tamil Nadu Forest Academy left a lasting impression on me. Our daily routine was structured as follows:

From Monday to Saturday, we had to assemble promptly at 5:45 am in front of our hostel, dressed uniformly in white attire and shoes, for a brisk one-and-a-half-hour session of rigorous physical training. Following this training, we would return to the hostel mess for a cup of tea or coffee.

Between 7:30 am and 8:45 am, we were allotted time for personal tasks such as bathing, laundry, room organization, and communicating with family and friends. Breakfast was also included in this period.

At 8:45 am, we would gather in front of the hostel and march towards the college building. Our day was packed with classes covering various subjects from 9 am to 4:15 pm, with a brief lunch break from 1:15 pm to 2 pm. Evening tea was served from 4:15 pm to 4:30 pm, followed by sports activities from 5 pm to 6:30 pm.

After returning from the sports ground, while some opted for baths and reading, a close colleague named Debo and I would head outside the campus to a tea shop. We would engage in extended discussions on a wide range of topics, including global and local issues, politics, history, culture, and more. This evening ritual lasted from 7:30 pm to 8:30 pm. Dinner was consumed between 8:30 pm and 9:00 pm, after which we all had to attend roll call at 9:00 pm to avoid any disciplinary actions.

Subsequently, some individuals played carrom, watched television, or retired to their rooms to sleep. This routine marked a stark departure from the lifestyle I had led in previous years. Over time, these practices became ingrained as habits.

The training also involved a phase at the Special Task Force (STF) training camp, nestled within the heart of a tiger reserve forest near the Moyer River. This camp offered only basic facilities such as tents for rest and a single camp tool that accompanied us for practical sessions in the forest. With no electricity, fencing, or boundaries, we were constantly alert, which provided a sense of thrill and a unique experience.

Basic toilets were located at a distance from the tents, requiring individuals to be accompanied by a peer when using them. Bathing and use of perfumes or soaps were strictly prohibited. The central kitchen area was illuminated by a single prominent light.

On our arrival at the training center in the evening, a startling event occurred. As we gathered at the center of the training camp, a tiger roared twice nearby. My initial thought was that the instructor was orchestrating a test of our courage in the forest. However, the instructor signaled us to remain silent and followed the roars toward the riverbank, attempting to locate the source. In the dimming light of the forest, it proved challenging to discern the tiger's whereabouts. As we waited, the tiger roared again, even closer this time, evoking fear among us. After a period of anticipation, we regrouped and received a briefing from the instructor on camp procedures and survival techniques.

Our training encompassed activities such as rope climbing, river crossings, wall climbing, combat training, and jungle survival. One remarkable experience involved a 25 km trek through hilly jungle terrain, culminating in an overnight stay at a village temple. This endeavor made me contemplate how much I had grown, considering that I once struggled with even simple tasks like using the bathroom.

A vital lesson I garnered from this experience was to remain prepared for potential danger without succumbing to anxiety. Being constantly prepared is essential, yet fixating on potential future events can render us more vulnerable. Instead, it's crucial to focus on readiness and immediate actions, always assessing the options available in any challenging situation:

A. If you possess the strength and capability to confront the challenge head-on, you're well-equipped.
B. If you lack the strength, invest effort to enhance your capabilities before the challenge arises.

This approach underscores the importance of proactive preparation and self-improvement, allowing us to face uncertainties with confidence and resilience.

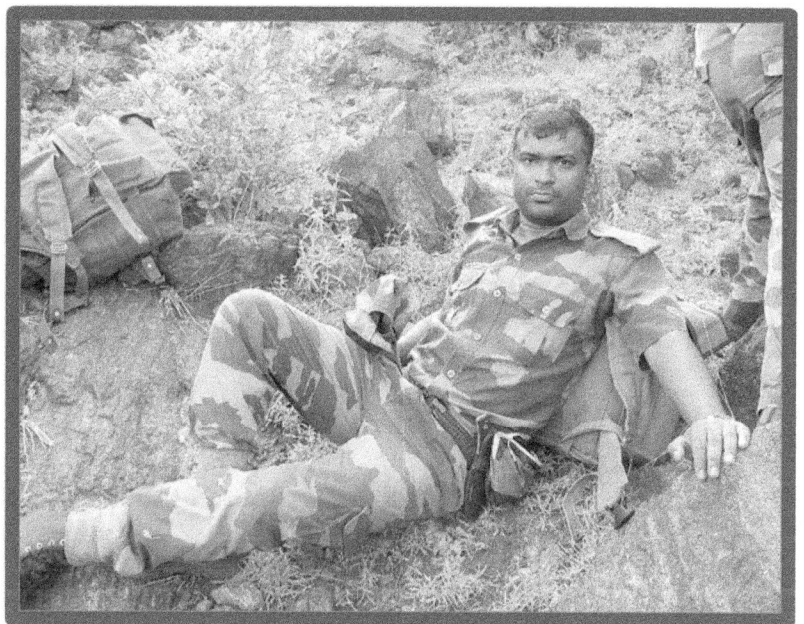

During Trekking Some Rest

CHAPTER NINE 9:

THE STORIES INSPIRE ME MOST:

"The beautiful thing about learning is nobody can take it away from you."—B.B. King

THE STORIES INSPIRE ME MOST:

Dashrath Manjhi : Dashrath Manjhi, often referred to as the Mountain Man, was a destitute laborer from Gehlaur village near Gaya in Bihar, India, born around 1934 and passing away on 17 August 2007. He achieved remarkable fame for his extraordinary endeavor of carving a passage through a hillock using only a hammer and chisel. This path measured 110 meters in length, 9.1 meters in width, and 7.6 meters in depth. His monumental work significantly shortened the travel distance between the Atri and Wazirganj blocks of Gaya town, reducing it from 55 kilometers to 15 kilometers.

Early in his life, Dashrath Manjhi fled his home and found employment in the coal mines of Dhanbad. Returning to his village, he married Falguni Devi. Tragedy struck when his wife, while bringing him lunch, suffered repeated falls on Gehlour hills, leading to serious injuries that ultimately resulted in her death. The loss deeply affected Manjhi, and that very night, he resolved to carve a path through the hills to facilitate better access to medical aid for his village. With unyielding determination, he meticulously chipped away at the Gehlour hills, creating a path that was 110 meters long, 7.7 meters deep in some areas, and 9.1 meters wide. In the face of skepticism and mockery, Manjhi remained unwavering, saying, "When I started hammering the hill, people called me a lunatic but that steeled my resolve."

The laborious project spanned 22 years, from 1960 to 1983. The path he carved significantly reduced the distance between the Atri and Wazirganj sectors of Gaya district, making life easier for the villagers. Despite initial ridicule, some villagers eventually extended support by providing food and helping him acquire tools.

Dashrath Manjhi passed away at the age of 73 on 17 August 2007 due to gall bladder cancer at the All India Institute of Medical Sciences (AIIMS) in New Delhi. His contributions earned him the nickname "Mountain Man." The Bihar government nominated him for the Padma Shree award in the social service sector in 2006. In honor of his legacy, India Post issued a stamp as part of the "Personalities of Bihar" series on 26 December 2016.

Karoly Takacs the man who won in olympics twice with his only hand:

Karoly Takacs is a name not widely recognized, yet he stands as a national hero in Hungary, celebrated for his remarkable story that exemplifies the indomitable strength of human willpower. His tale serves as a profound testament to the incredible potential that lies within the human spirit.

In the year 1938, Karoly Takacs, a member of the Hungarian Army, held the prestigious title of the world's foremost pistol shooter. His sights were set on capturing the gold medal at the upcoming 1940 Olympic Games in Tokyo, a feat that seemed well within his grasp.

However, fate took a devastating turn mere months before the Olympics. During a training exercise with his army unit, an unfortunate incident occurred – a hand grenade explosion robbed Takacs of his right hand, effectively snuffing out his dreams of Olympic glory.

In the wake of this tragic event, Takacs faced a pivotal crossroads, with his aspirations hanging in the balance. Despite the odds, he was left with two options:

Relinquish his pursuit of shooting: This would have been the easiest path, with sympathy and understanding expected from all corners.

Forge ahead with the dream using his left hand: Instead of fixating on his loss, he chose to focus on his potential.

Following the accident, Takacs found himself spending a month in the hospital, grappling with both the loss of his hand and the demise of his Olympic aspirations. For most, this juncture would have marked the end of the journey, a point of no return. Yet, Takacs was not an ordinary individual; he was a winner. Winners understand that adversity cannot define them, and that life's challenges cannot deter them. They possess an unshakable conviction that quitting is simply not an option.

With uncommon determination, Takacs refused to be defeated. He rose from the ashes of despair, resolved to learn the art of shooting with his left hand. He posed a simple question to himself: "Why not?" Rather than lamenting his missing right hand, he chose to concentrate on his incredible mental strength and the potential of his healthy left hand, envisioning its transformation into a champion's tool through dedicated effort.

In the solitude of his practice, Takacs toiled for months, keeping his endeavors hidden from the world. Perhaps he sought to shield himself from the discouragement he might have encountered had his renewed pursuit been public knowledge.

In the spring of 1939, he unveiled his newfound skill at the Hungarian National Pistol Shooting Championship. Fellow competitors approached him with condolences and admiration for his resolve to attend the event despite his circumstances. Their surprise was palpable when Takacs declared, "I didn't come to watch; I came to compete." And to their greater astonishment, he emerged victorious.

The 1940 and 1944 Olympics were canceled due to World War II, threatening to forever shatter Takacs' Olympic aspirations. Nonetheless, Takacs persevered, training diligently, and in 1948, he qualified for the London Olympics. While his peers competed with both hands intact, Takacs faced the challenge with only one hand. At the age of 38, he secured the Gold Medal and set a new world record in pistol shooting. His triumph continued four years later at the 1952 Helsinki Olympics, as he claimed the Gold Medal once again. Takacs, a paragon of mental resilience, triumphed against all odds.

In contrast, a loser is quick to furnish an array of excuses, citing myriad reasons for failure. A winner, however, identifies a single reason why they can succeed. Winners habitually choose to perceive even the faintest glimmers of positivity and say to themselves, "That's alright. A solution exists, and I will unearth it."

The swift pace of Takacs' recovery was crucial to maintaining his momentum and drive. In a mere month, he managed to rebound from his predicament. Had he wallowed in his despair or succumbed to his circumstances, relinquishing the pursuit of excellence, he would have forfeited the keen edge of his determination. His resilience, his "eye of the tiger," would have dulled, preventing him from making a triumphant return.

Takacs had every right to yield to his despair and ask, "Why me?" perpetually. He could have succumbed to mediocrity, allowing the accident to shroud him in despondency and resignation. He could have adopted the posture of a loser.

Yet, Takacs opted for a different path. He chose to delve into the depths of his being, uncovering a solution rather than succumbing to his challenges. He resolved to pick himself up and master the art of shooting anew. Winners, like Takacs, are driven by a relentless pursuit of solutions, while losers seek refuge in excuses.

The next time you find yourself knocked down by life's challenges, make the choice to respond as a winner. Adopt Takacs' mindset, rise swiftly, take action, and astonish the world with your resolve.

CHAPTER TEN 10:

THE PC GAME CHANGE MY PERCEPTION ABOUT MY LIFE:

"Laziness erodes a person of his enthusiasm and energy. As a result the person loses all opportunities and finally becomes dejected and frustrated. The worst thing is that he stops believing in himself." – Sam Veda

THE PC GAME CHANGE MY PERCEPTION ABOUT MY LIFE:

Amidst my moments of suffering, when television failed to captivate my attention, I sought solace in the realm of PC gaming. Real-time strategy games, in particular, held a special allure for me. This preference was largely shaped by the geographical distance of my city from the bustling capital, a circumstance that made procuring recent and high-quality games a rare and arduous endeavor. Unfortunately, the local game shop owners exhibited scant interest in catering to the niche of real-time strategy enthusiasts, as the demand was limited. Despite these challenges, I managed to amass a modest collection of these games.

During one ordinary day, I chanced upon a newspaper review of a game named "SIM." Instantly, its premise captured my imagination. However, my excitement was short-lived as I scoured the local market in vain for this elusive game. Frustration welled within me, tinged with a glimmer of hope that someday I might experience the game that had intrigued me.

Then, a ray of hope emerged when my brother returned from the market, triumphantly bearing the coveted game "SIM." Our shared enthusiasm was palpable as we reveled in the realization that the elusive game was now within our grasp. I beheld my desire incarnate, nestled in my brother's hands, and an overwhelming sense of joy flooded over me.

For those unfamiliar with the game, "The Sims 2" is a strategic life simulation video game developed by Maxis and published by Electronic

Arts in 2004. It follows the legacy of its predecessor, "The Sims." The gameplay centers on guiding virtual characters, or "Sims," through various life stages, from infancy to old age, and managing their aspirations, relationships, and daily activities.

In my gaming escapades, a recurring pattern emerged. As I delved into the immersive world of "The Sims 2," I found myself engrossed in creating and shaping characters that mirrored my own persona. My digital alter ego, named RAJ, embodied my aspirations and desires within the game. My primary objective was to accumulate wealth and construct opulent abodes, a process that I found particularly enthralling. The act of crafting elaborate dwellings became an unexpected form of entertainment, allowing me to explore architectural creativity.

Opting for the role of a shrewd businessman, I diligently pursued the accumulation of virtual wealth. Yet, managing my virtual character's well-being proved to be a challenge. Despite my intention to make decisions that would lead to success, my character, akin to a stubborn entity, sometimes resisted my guidance. I could predict his desires and needs more acutely than he could himself. It was a perplexing realization to recognize that while playing, I perceived myself as the omnipotent force shaping his life.

However, a revelation struck me one day while engrossed in the game. I instructed my virtual counterpart to swiftly ascend the ladder of success, aiming to accrue substantial wealth for the construction of an extravagant mansion. But to my bewilderment, he resisted my commands, his mood plummeting as he demanded expensive items and rest. This internal conflict mirrored my own struggle to adhere to divine guidance while seeking my personal comfort zone.

A profound insight unfurled within my mind: I had been the ignorant fool, obstinately resisting the divine instructions for five to seven years. The very act of complaining to a higher power for aid, while ensnared in the cocoon of my comfort zone, echoed my virtual character's defiance.

This realization initiated a transformative journey. I ventured into the realm of meditation, a practice that led me to experience a heightened connection with the divine instructions that had eluded me for so long. Gradually, I began to feel the divine guidance coursing through me, imparting strength and wisdom. This profound shift in perspective prompted me to abandon my self-imposed boundaries and follow the divine will.

My experience : My experience while playing the game was a fascinating exploration of both virtual realms and profound self-realization. With each session, I would create a character and inevitably name him "RAJ," a reflection of myself in this digital universe. The underlying purpose of my gameplay was multifaceted: my primary goal was to accumulate wealth diligently, while also indulging in the creative pursuit of constructing grand and exquisite houses. Designing these virtual homes emerged as an unexpectedly delightful aspect of the game, one that resonated deeply with me and ignited my passion.

Within the virtual realm, I charted the course of my character's life, akin to molding my own destiny. My aspiration was clear: to ascend the ranks as a shrewd businessman, amassing riches with agility. This pursuit, while digital, mirrored my own ambition for financial growth in the real world.

Yet, controlling my virtual counterpart proved to be a nuanced challenge. As I navigated his daily existence, striving to fulfill his needs and desires, I was reminded of the intricate dance between individual desires and external influences. It became evident that I understood the inner workings of this virtual persona, "RAJ," more intricately than he understood himself.

My decisions for him were meticulously curated, designed to ensure his prosperity and well-being. However, as if to defy my careful planning, he occasionally rebelled. He would make unexpected demands, clamoring for entertainment or costly acquisitions, and at times even insisting on rest. In these moments, I found myself in the role of a digital deity, orchestrating the destiny of my virtual creation. As I wielded the power to shape his life, I was reminded of the parallels between my role in the game and the greater cosmic forces guiding our lives.

Then came a pivotal day within the digital narrative. I resolved to propel my virtual counterpart toward new heights by mastering a particular skill, a step toward realizing his dream of becoming a successful businessman. Additionally, I harbored a grand vision of amassing substantial wealth to construct a sprawling mansion—a dream home worthy of his aspirations. The construction aspect of the game, where I could meticulously design and build his residence, enthralled me deeply.

However, in a twist that mirrored life's unpredictability, my virtual character defied my intentions. His virtual mood took a dip, and he began demanding opulent items—an expensive TV set, a lavish sofa, and even rest. Frustration surged within me, prompting an exasperated thought: "Why doesn't he follow my directives?"

It was in this moment that a spark of profound realization ignited within my mind. An epiphany dawned upon me, revealing a startling truth. I was no different from my digital alter ego, "RAJ." I had been ensnared in my own cocoon of comfort, resisting the divine guidance that sought to shape my life's journey. I had spent years resisting divine wisdom, much like my virtual character resisted my guidance in the game.

The analogy was striking. How many times had I, through self-imposed limitations, bound myself in invisible threads of fear and comfort? How often had I cried out to a higher power, questioning why I wasn't being rescued from my self-created quagmire? It was a humbling realization that shook me to my core.

In the aftermath of this revelation, a newfound path beckoned. I embarked on a journey of meditation, seeking to quiet my mind and connect with the divine guidance that had eluded me for so long. Gradually, as I tuned into this higher wisdom, I felt a strengthening of spirit. I learned to trust in myself and in the divine intelligence that permeates all of existence.

In closing, my venture into the virtual world of "The Sims 2" unraveled a profound lesson that resonated far beyond the confines of the game. Just as my virtual counterpart resisted my guidance, I had resisted divine guidance in my life. This revelation propelled me toward a transformative journey of self-discovery and spiritual connection. I learned that embracing divine wisdom entails transcending self-imposed limitations and trusting the unseen forces that understand us better than we understand ourselves.

CHAPTER ELEVEN 11:

ALL INSTRUCTIONS IN BRIEF:

"When there is harmony between the mind, heart, and resolution, then nothing is impossible." – Rig Veda

ALL INSTRUCTIONS IN BRIEF:

Embarking on a journey of self-improvement and personal growth is akin to embarking on a grand adventure. Just as in any journey, it's perfectly alright not to tackle all the challenges or practices at once. In fact, this gradual approach is often the most effective and sustainable way to bring about meaningful change in your life.

Consider it as if you're constructing a complex puzzle. Each piece of the puzzle represents a practice or task that contributes to your personal growth and well-being. You don't need to rush to fit all the pieces together in one go. Instead, you can select the pieces that resonate with you the most and start piecing them together at a pace that feels comfortable.

It's understandable if the idea of implementing numerous changes all at once feels overwhelming. Life is already filled with commitments, responsibilities, and daily routines. Adding too many new practices in one go might lead to burnout or a sense of being stretched too thin.

By choosing to take it one step at a time, you're ensuring that you can fully absorb and integrate each practice into your life. Imagine that you're planting seeds in a garden. Each seed represents a practice you want to incorporate. Planting too many seeds at once might lead to uneven growth and inadequate attention to each seed's development. On the other hand, when you plant one seed, nurture it, and watch it flourish, you're setting a strong foundation for the next seed you'll plant.

Start with the practices that feel accessible and manageable. Perhaps you choose to start your day with a brief meditation or dedicate a few minutes to journaling before bed. As you begin to experience the positive impact of these practices, you'll naturally feel motivated to expand your efforts.

The beauty of this gradual approach is that it allows you to customize your journey. You can adapt the practices to your unique lifestyle, schedule, and preferences. As you slowly incorporate each practice, you're building a foundation of positive habits that will support you over time.

It's also important to acknowledge that change takes time. Just as you can't rush the growth of a plant, you can't rush your personal development. By focusing on incremental progress, you're giving yourself the gift of patience and self-compassion.

Remember that the journey is just as valuable as the destination. Embrace the process of self-discovery, growth, and transformation. Each step you take, no matter how small, brings you closer to the vision of the person you aspire to become. So, take your time, enjoy the journey, and celebrate the victories—big and small—along the way.

MEDICINAL PLANTS.

"Do not harm the man who digs you up, nor him for whom nor I dig you up; let all our two footed and four-footed creatures be without sickness" ………..*Line from the most famous hymn is the 'THE HEALING PLANTS' hymn in Rig Veda (10-97).*

These three herbs—*Ocimum sanctum* (Holy Basil), *Bacopa monnieri* (Brahmi), and *Centella asiatica*—are nature's gifts that have been revered for their profound effects on reducing anxiety and depression. Incorporating these herbs into your daily routine can bring about significant improvements in mental well-being.

Ocimum sanctum (Holy Basil):

Holy Basil, also known as *Ocimum sanctum* or Tulsi, holds a special place in traditional medicine and cultural practices. Its ability to soothe racing thoughts and alleviate anxiety is truly remarkable. Consuming 5 to 10 leaves of Holy Basil daily has shown to be effective in calming the mind and promoting a sense of tranquility. Beyond its anxiety-relieving properties, Holy Basil boasts an array of health benefits. It possesses antimicrobial, adaptogenic, anti-inflammatory, and immune-modulating properties. Considered sacred by Hindus, this herb has been a part of rituals and practices for generations. While some may consider it a superstition, its rich medicinal value and adaptogenic properties have made it a staple for those seeking natural remedies for anxiety and overall well-being.

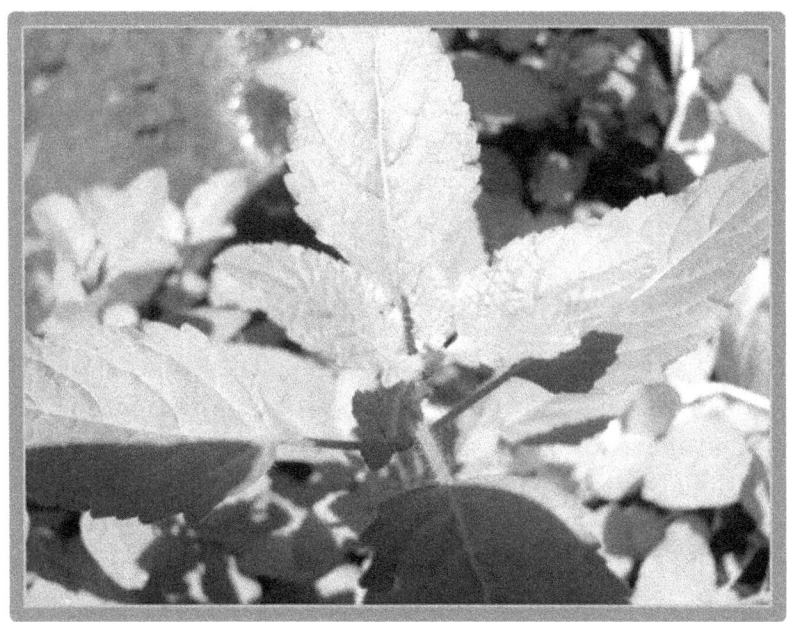

Ocimum sanctum (Holy Basil):

Bacopa monnieri (Brahmi):

Bacopa monnieri, commonly referred to as Brahmi, has a profound impact on cognitive health. Not only does it reduce anxiety, but it also enhances memory and cognitive function. This herb interacts with dopamine and serotonergic systems, contributing to its anxiety-reducing effects. Brahmi has a historical significance in Ayurvedic medicine, where it is recognized for its memory-enhancing properties. It's worth noting that "Brahmi" has been used to refer to two different herbs—*Bacopa monnieri* and *Centella asiatica*. To make the consumption of bitter *Bacopa monnieri* more palatable, innovative methods can be employed.

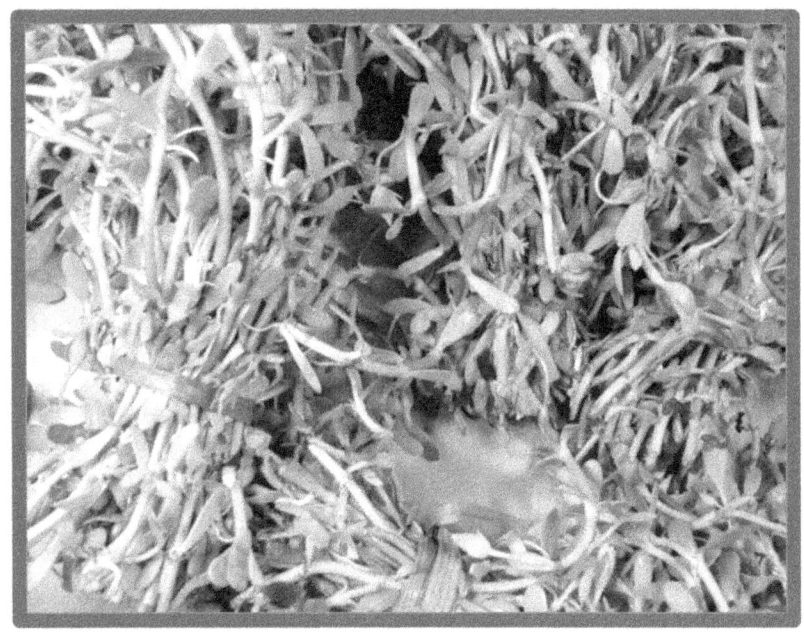

Bacopa monnieri or (Brahmi)

***Centella asiatica*:**

Centella asiatica, also known as Gotu Kola, holds a prominent place as a rejuvenating herb in Ayurvedic medicine. Its leaves are believed to promote longevity and peaceful sleep while combating stress and depression. By energizing the central nervous system and replenishing energy reserves, *Centella asiatica* acts as a natural tonic for mental well-being. Consuming one to two leaves on an empty stomach in the morning has been advocated by certain Hindu religious groups. Their practices align with the herb's reputation for enhancing reflexes, increasing libido, and preventing nervous breakdowns.

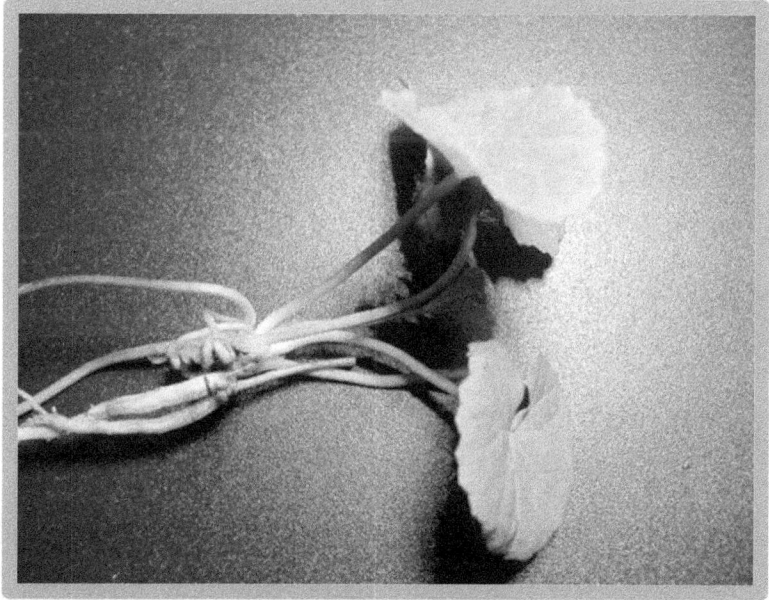

Centella asiatica

Incorporating these herbs into your routine is not just a matter of health—it's a way of connecting with centuries-old wisdom and traditions that recognized the power of nature in healing the mind and body. Just as you elaborate on the various properties of these herbs, remember that their benefits go beyond their physiological effects. They carry a legacy of holistic well-being that intertwines nature, culture, and the human experience.

Transforming the consumption of Bitter Bacopa monnieri into a pleasurable experience: Given the notably bitter taste of Brahmi or Bacopa monnieri, incorporating it into one's daily routine was indeed a challenge. However, I innovatively turned this into an enjoyable habit by finding a way to make its consumption delicious on a daily basis.

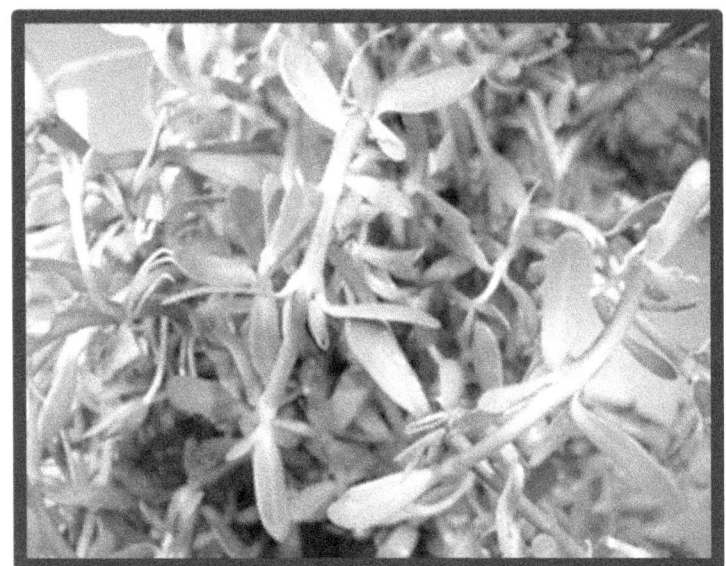

A. Collect or buy Bacopa monnieri.

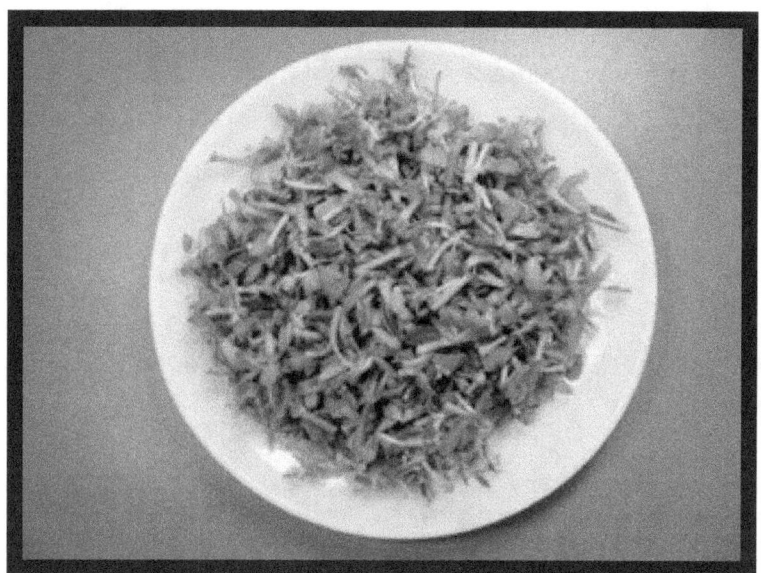

B.   Cut into small pieces.

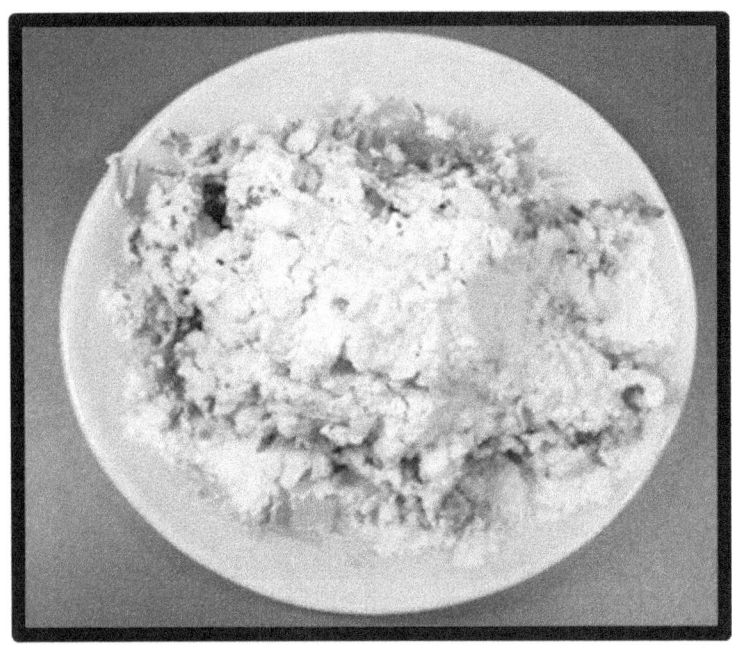

C. Add some besan or Gram flour /garbanzo bean flour/chickpea flour and salt.

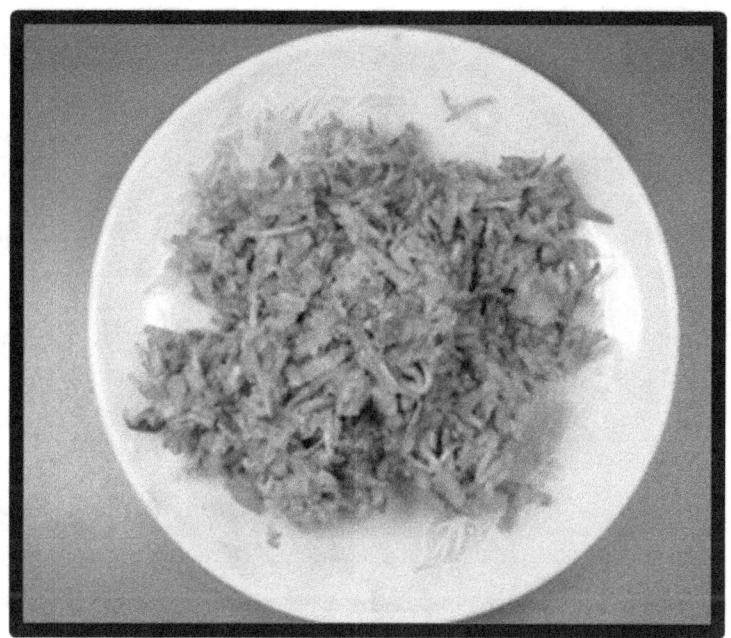

D. Add very small amount water and mix all.

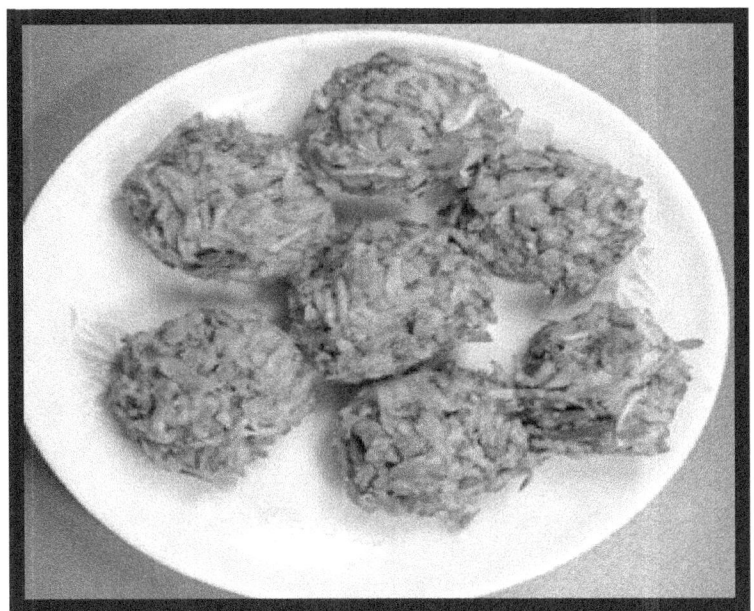

E. Make round shape.

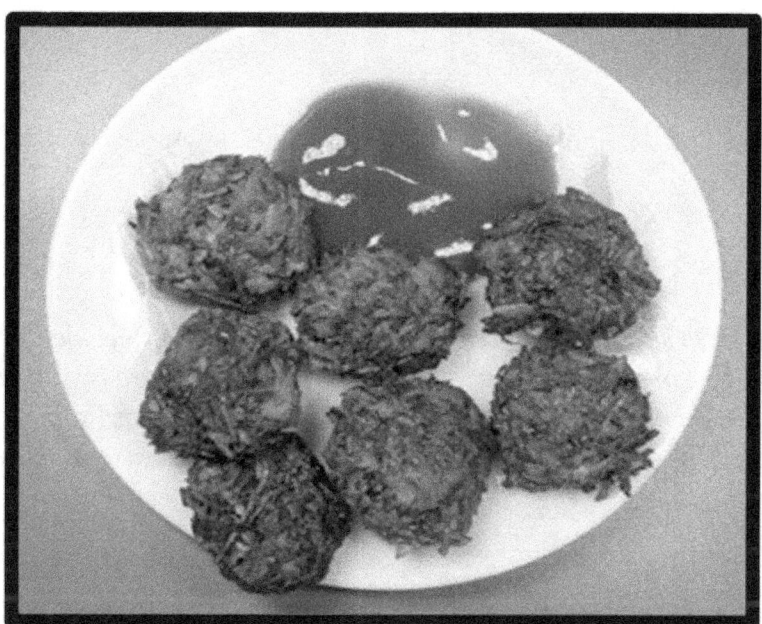

F. Heat oil in a frying pan and fry them and eat with tomato sauce.

[In case these specific herbs are not readily available in your local area, you might encounter difficulty finding them. However, there is a solution: several e-commerce platforms offer dried leaves of these herbs for purchase. This option allows you to access their benefits even if sourcing them locally is a challenge.]

MEDITATION (SIMPLE AND EFFECTIVE MEDITATION TECHNIQUE)

"Do not be led by others,awaken your own mind,amass your own experience,and decide for yourself your own path."— **Veda**

Achieving Effective Meditation Without Prior Practice or Skills:

Meditation can often seem like a challenging endeavor, especially for those of us who are not seasoned yogis residing in the serene Himalayan Mountains. The demands of our modern lives, coupled with our racing thoughts, lack of concentration, and stress-ridden minds, can make learning meditation a daunting task. However, I have discovered a simple meditation technique that offers tangible results right from the very first day, even for beginners.

Here is a step-by-step guide to this approach:

Step 1: Gather Your Equipment

Obtain a pair of high-quality earplugs and place them snugly in your ears. Following this, put on a well-fitting earmuff over your ears. By doing so, you effectively create a soundproof barrier between yourself and the external world. This is essential for creating a calm and distraction-free environment for your meditation session.

Step 2: Set Your Intentions

Before you begin, make an unbreakable commitment to yourself that you will not allow any thoughts to intrude upon your meditation. This intention will lay the foundation for your practice.

Step 3: Breathing and Counting

With your earplugs and earmuffs in place, take a deep breath in and start counting down from 10 to 0. Breathe slowly and steadily with each count. This rhythmic breathing helps calm your mind and prepare it for the meditation exercise.

Step 4: Listen to Inner Sounds

As you reach the count of 0, shift your focus to your inner world. Try to listen intently to the subtle, continuous inner sound that naturally exists within you. This sound can be likened to a gentle and soothing "zzzzzzzzzzzzzzzzzzzzz." Allow yourself to be fully immersed in this internal auditory experience.

Step 5: Choose the Right Timing

It is advisable to practice this meditation technique before going to sleep. By doing so, you create a serene mental state that significantly contributes to achieving deep and restful sleep. This technique facilitates the kind of rejuvenating sleep that revitalizes not only your mind but also your body and brain cells.

Step 6: Share the Technique

Recognize the effectiveness of this meditation method and share it with your family members and friends. Its simplicity and immediate benefits make it accessible to individuals from all walks of life.

Incorporating this technique into your routine can bring about a profound positive impact on your mental well-being, helping you achieve a sense of tranquility even amidst the challenges of everyday life. This meditation approach offers a gateway to a refreshing sleep, which, in turn, aids in the rejuvenation of both

your mind and body.

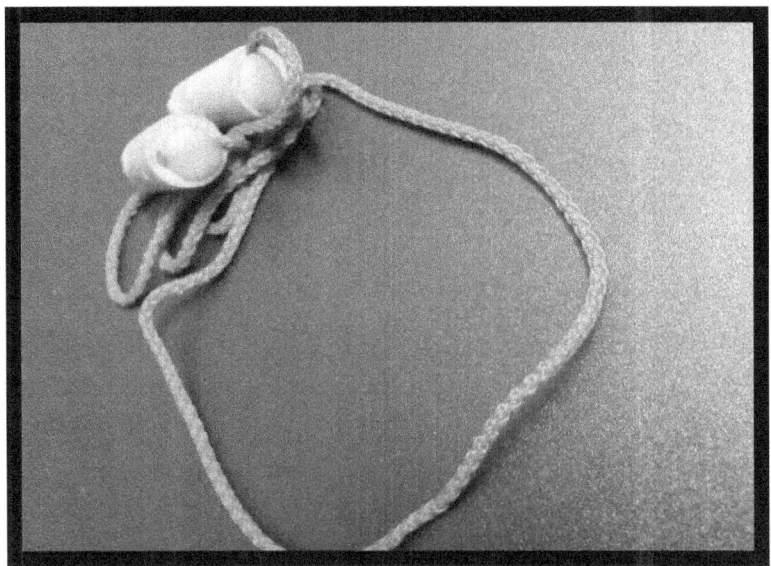

Ear Plug

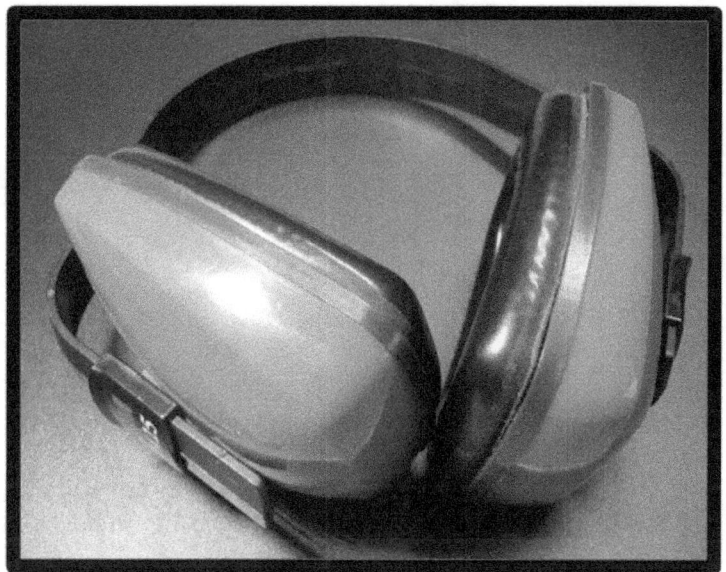

Ear Muff

EXERCISE AND YOGA.

"Knowing Him who is the origin and dissolution of the universe – the source of all virtue, the destroyer of all sins, the master of all good qualities, the immortal, and the abode of the universe – as seated in one's own self, He is perceived as different from, and transcending, the tree of Samsara as well as time and form."– Shvetashvatara Upanishad

Exercise and Yoga are pivotal in the battle against anxiety and depression. Personally, I procured a manual treadmill machine to integrate a daily workout routine into my life. In the initial stages, my sessions were brief – I would stand on the treadmill for just 10 minutes. My body and mind were yet to synchronize with the notion of consistent walking. Gradually, I advanced to walking for the same 10-minute duration and, over time, escalated it to a fulfilling hour. The impact of exercise was nothing short of transformative – it not only helped restore my self-assurance but also fostered holistic well-being, effectively mitigating my anxiety and depression.

The mechanism behind exercise's efficacy is rooted in the intricate interplay of hormones, with Brain-Derived Neurotrophic Factor (BDNF) taking center stage. BDNF, a critical neurotransmitter, facilitates the generation of new brain cells, thereby aiding cognitive health. Another vital element of exercise is the release of endorphins, often referred to as the body's natural "feel-good" chemicals. These endorphins engage with specialized receptors in the brain, known as opioid receptors, to reduce pain perception while also inducing a sense of positivity akin to that prompted by morphine. These endorphins function as both pain alleviators and gratification inducers, forging a compelling incentive to engage in regular exercise for at least 30 minutes.

Complementing my exercise regimen was the practice of Yoga, which played an equally significant role in my journey to recovery. My daily routine incorporated fundamental yoga postures and three specific Pranayama techniques, which collectively contributed to alleviating my condition.

A. Anulom Vilom Pranayama:

Anulom Vilom Pranayama involves a simple yet effective sequence. Begin by closing your eyes and assuming the Padmasana posture, with your hands resting on your knees. Proceed to seal your right nostril with your thumb and gently inhale through your left nostril, ensuring a deliberate, unhurried inhalation until your lungs are completely filled. Next, release your right nostril and exhale. With your middle finger, occlude your left nostril as you inhale through your right nostril. Following this, employ your thumb to seal your right nostril again and exhale through your left nostril. This rhythmic alternation should be repeated for 5 to 10 minutes, focusing intently on your breath and gradually increasing the practice duration as proficiency builds.

B. Sitali Pranayama:

Sitali Pranayama is practiced while seated in the Easy Pose, maintaining an upright spine. Begin by curling your tongue and extending it slightly beyond your lips. Inhale deeply through your mouth and tongue, experiencing a cooling sensation in your mouth and throat as the air courses through. This breath should be directed into your belly, allowing it to expand fully. As you exhale, utilize your nose. This soothing process can be repeated for 2 to 5 minutes, with the option to extend the duration as you become more adept.

C. Suryaved Pranayama:

For Suryaved Pranayama, assume a comfortable asana of your choice. Block your left nostril with the ring finger of your right hand. Inhale deeply through your right nostril, holding the breath within your lungs for 10 seconds. Subsequently, use your right thumb to close your right nostril and exhale through your left nostril. This sequence can be repeated for 2 to 3 minutes, adjusting the duration as your familiarity with the practice grows.

These Pranayama techniques, in conjunction with consistent exercise, constituted an indispensable component of my healing journey. Over the course of months, I observed their cumulative impact on my mental well-being, underscoring the significance of these practices as holistic tools for managing anxiety and depression.

FRUITS AND NUTRITION.

"O, parna mani! You are a leaf, but you are the protector of my body. May you increase my valour. I will wear your energy on my person for an entire year…………………….. Atharvana Veda

Providing your brain and body with a nourishing and balanced diet is essential for optimal functioning. Certain foods are particularly beneficial in supporting your overall health. Consider incorporating the following items into your daily meals:

Walnuts: Rich in omega-3 fatty acids, antioxidants, and vitamins, walnuts are known to promote brain health and support cognitive function. These nutrients contribute to improved memory and focus, making walnuts a valuable addition to your diet.

Almonds: Soaking and blending almonds can enhance their nutrient absorption. Almonds offer a source of healthy fats, vitamin E, and essential minerals. These nutrients play a role in maintaining brain health, aiding nerve communication, and supporting overall well-being.

Sweet Figs: Figs are a natural source of dietary fiber, vitamins, and minerals. Their natural sweetness makes them a satisfying alternative to sugary snacks. The fiber content supports digestive health and helps stabilize blood sugar levels, contributing to steady energy throughout the day.

Dry Coconut: Coconut contains medium-chain triglycerides (MCTs), which are easily metabolized by the body and can provide a quick source of energy. Additionally, coconut offers essential nutrients that support various bodily functions.

Dates: Dates are rich in natural sugars, fiber, and essential minerals like potassium and magnesium. They provide a quick energy boost and can help prevent energy crashes between meals. The fiber content aids in digestion and supports a healthy gut.

Flax Seeds: Flax seeds are particularly noteworthy due to their high content of omega-3 fatty acids, specifically alpha-linolenic acid (ALA). These fatty acids are crucial for brain health and have been linked to reduced risk of depression and improved mood. Grinding flax seeds before consumption enhances nutrient absorption, and a light dry roasting process can enhance their flavor and nutritional value.

Research has shown that individuals with depression often have lower levels of docosahexaenoic acid (DHA) and eicosapentaenoic acid (EPA), which are types of omega-3 fatty acids. These acids are abundant in foods like fatty fish, walnuts, and flax seeds. By incorporating these foods into your diet, you're providing your body with the essential building blocks for maintaining emotional well-being and cognitive function.

Remember that a balanced diet should also include a variety of other nutrient-rich foods such as vegetables, fruits, whole grains, lean proteins, and healthy fats. Consulting with a healthcare professional or registered dietitian can help you create a personalized nutrition plan that meets your specific needs and health goals.

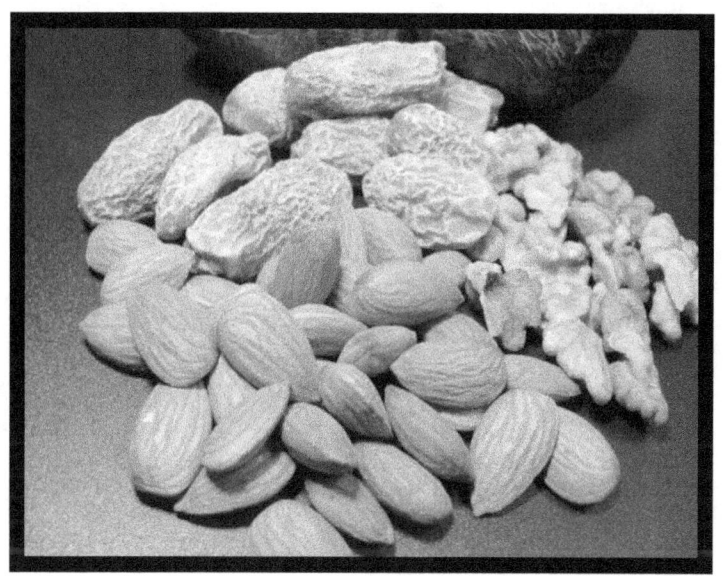

Essential Nuts

WHAT YOU MUST AVOID

"Avoidance is a wonderful therapy" — Maggie Stiefvater, Linger

Taking care of your mental and emotional well-being involves making conscious choices about your daily activities and interactions. Here are some guidelines to consider for a healthier mindset:

Limit Social Networking: It's advisable to take a break from social networking activities for around 6 to 7 months or until you feel you've made substantial progress, reaching around 70% to 80% of your recovery. Finding happiness solely through uploading pictures or videos can be counterproductive to your well-being. Similarly, avoid the urge to constantly check others' profiles, as this behavior can lead to unhappiness and comparison.

Reduce TV Time: While television might have initially seemed like a solution to your problems, it can turn into a source of anxiety, depression, and fear. The constant barrage of sensory stimuli, including sound and images, can overwhelm your mind and prevent you from properly addressing your challenges. An overstimulated mind can also ruminate on problems during shows. Limiting your TV time allows your brain to focus on more constructive activities.

Avoid Alcohol and Drugs: While you mention that you're not addicted, it's still important to keep alcohol consumption to a minimum and steer clear of other drugs. Substance use can have negative effects on mental health, exacerbating anxiety and depression. By maintaining a sober lifestyle, you're better positioned to manage your emotions and challenges.

Surround Yourself with Positivity: Choose to spend time with people who have a positive and optimistic outlook on life. Negative and pessimistic individuals can drain your energy and contribute to your own negative feelings. Also, be mindful of the content you consume. Limit exposure to negative news and topics that you have no control over, as these can heighten feelings of helplessness and anxiety.

Mindful Consumption of Media: Watching pornography before bedtime can disrupt your sleep patterns and impact your overall well-being. It's recommended to avoid such content before sleep to ensure a more restful and restorative rest.

Taking these steps can contribute to a more balanced and positive mental state. However, remember that everyone's journey is unique. It's important to tailor these guidelines to your specific circumstances and consult with a mental health professional if you're facing significant challenges. Their guidance can provide personalized strategies to support your recovery and well-being.

WHAT YOU MUST DO

Don't just learn, experience.
Don't just read, absorb.
Don't just change, transform.
Don't just relate, advocate.
Don't just promise, prove.
Don't just criticize, encourage.
Don't just think, ponder.
Don't just take, give.
Don't just see, feel.
Don't just dream, do.
Don't just hear, listen.
Don't just talk, act.
Don't just tell, show.
Don't just exist, live."
— Roy T. Bennett, The Light in the Heart

Engaging in a set of positive routines and activities can greatly contribute to your mental well-being. Here's a detailed rephrasing of your suggestions:

Bedtime Reading Ritual: Cultivate a healthy bedtime routine to promote better sleep and relaxation. Spend around 30 minutes engrossed in a physical book before sleep. Avoid electronic devices and LED table lamps as they can disrupt sleep patterns. By engaging in this analog reading practice, you're allowing your mind to unwind and prepare for rest.

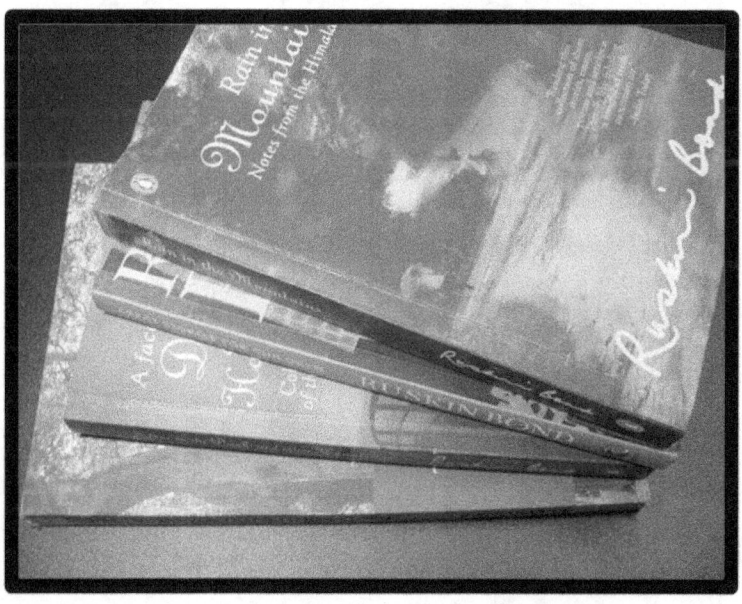

Mindful Music Listening: While music can have varying effects on mood, personalizing your music choices can yield positive results. Despite receiving advice to listen to music for mood elevation and anxiety reduction, you discovered that focusing on the lyrics sometimes had a negative impact. To counter this, you explored music in languages you're

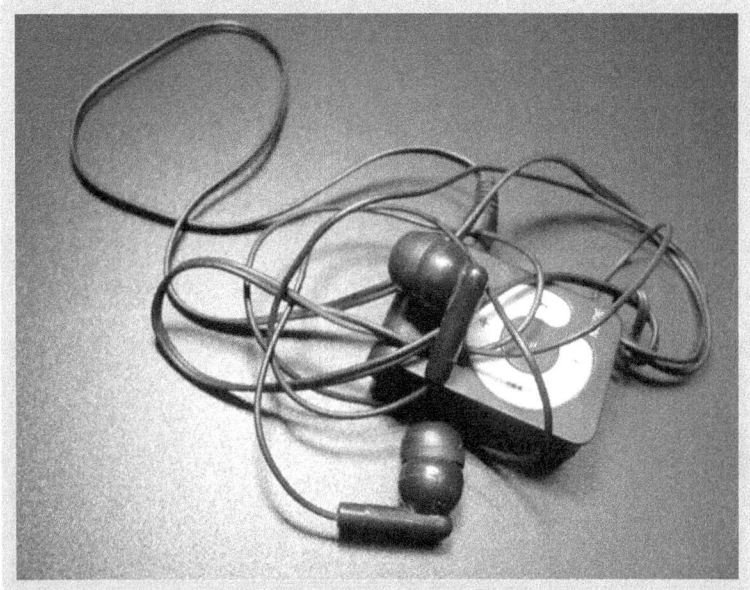

not familiar with, like Russian and Telugu. By immersing yourself in these songs, you successfully diverted your mind from anxious thoughts. It's important not to overindulge in music throughout the day.

Nature Connection: Spending time in nature has proven benefits for mental health, but there are creative ways to achieve this even when circumstances make it challenging. During a particularly difficult period of anxiety, you devised a method to trick your brain into a positive state by viewing downloaded nature wallpapers on your devices. These images acted as a visual escape, helping you recover quicker from stress. Incorporating this practice into your daily routine can provide regular boosts of positivity.

Motivational Reading: Inspirational literature can significantly impact your mindset. Consider reading motivational books or compiling a collection of 100 inspirational quotes that resonate with you. Having these quotes readily available offers a quick remedy when you're feeling down, helping you regain a more positive outlook.

Physical Activity: Regular exercise is a non-negotiable activity for your well-being. Dedicate time to exercise regularly, without allowing excuses to deter you. Physical activity has a profound impact on mental health, releasing endorphins that contribute to improved mood and overall vitality.

Diversify Your Sources of Happiness: Avoid relying solely on one source for your happiness. Instead, diversify your interests and engage in various activities. Exploring new hobbies, caring for an aquarium, spending quality time with your family, and extending kindness to others are effective ways to broaden your sources of happiness and boost your self-confidence.

Remember that these practices are personal to you and tailored to your experiences. While they have proven beneficial, everyone's journey is unique. If you find yourself struggling or facing persistent challenges, seeking guidance from a mental health professional is a crucial step toward achieving lasting well-being.

Engaging in the process of learning a new language can unexpectedly yield significant benefits for reducing anxiety and phobia. While I was personally grappling with these challenges, I discovered that my unintentional journey into learning Japanese and Spanish offered me a path toward relief. This realization was reinforced when I read about the positive impact of language acquisition on mental well-being in a newspaper. This discovery brought a sense of happiness and gratitude.

Learning a new language has been scientifically proven to be one of the most effective and pragmatic methods for enhancing intelligence, maintaining cognitive sharpness, and shielding the brain against the effects of aging. Remarkably, many individuals from India are adept in two, three, or even four languages – the native tongue, the national language Hindi, and often English. (It's worth noting that India boasts a remarkable 22 official languages, with around 150 languages spoken by sizable populations according to the Census of India.)

Further exploration online unveiled the myriad advantages of being bilingual or multilingual. Research has demonstrated that individuals proficient in multiple languages experience superior cognitive capabilities compared to monolingual counterparts. Those who speak more than one language are more likely to:

Demonstrate heightened general intelligence.

Excel in tasks related to planning, prioritization, and decision-making.

Achieve elevated scores in standardized assessments of mathematics, reading, and vocabulary.

Display enhanced empathy and the ability to comprehend differing perspectives.

Showcase improved concentration, focus, and attention.

Significantly, the act of acquiring a foreign language can contribute to the expansion of the brain's linguistic center and the hippocampus – a region responsible for memory formation, retention, and retrieval. This pivotal insight underscores the cognitive advantages associated with language learning.

To embark on this journey, I found the Duolingo app to be an invaluable resource. This online and mobile platform offers free lessons in vocabulary and fundamental grammar for beginners. By establishing personalized language learning goals within the Duolingo app, anyone can initiate their linguistic exploration and begin reaping the benefits.

In conclusion, the pursuit of acquiring a new language holds unexpected rewards for mitigating anxiety and phobia. Not only does it contribute to cognitive enhancement and mental resilience, but it also aligns with the natural multilingual capabilities of diverse populations. Through tools like Duolingo, this path to personal growth and mental well-being becomes easily accessible.

DISCLAIMER AND CAUTION:

Important Note:

It's essential to acknowledge that these suggestions are not intended to replace or substitute professional advice from medical practitioners or experts. Consultation with them remains paramount for comprehensive guidance.

Mindfulness During Practice:

Following a period of dedicated practice, typically lasting one to two weeks, it's common for an anxious or depressive mind to voice negative thoughts such as, "You can't let us go; we define you," or "Without us, you're insignificant and your existence is meaningless." Sometimes, these thoughts might create an internal void or emptiness. However, it's crucial not to heed their influence. Counter them resolutely and decisively. Through this process, you'll come to realize your distinct and formidable identity, separate from the grip of anxiety, fear, depression, or stress.

Gradual Progress and Acknowledgment:

Progress in your journey towards well-being should not be rushed. It's important to savor and appreciate even the smallest of improvements. Rather than expecting overnight transformations, embracing each incremental step forward allows for a more sustainable and fulfilling path to recovery.

Personal Photography:

Each image featured is a product of my personal photography, offering a genuine visual representation of the concepts presented.

Please remember that while these insights offer practical guidance, the expertise and guidance of medical professionals should always be prioritized, especially in matters concerning mental health. The struggle against negative thoughts and emotions is an ongoing process that requires patience, determination, and, at times, professional assistance.

--END--